# THE CANNABIS BASICS

## THE HISTORY, USAGE, CULTIVATION AND MEDICINAL BENEFITS OF THE CANNABIS PLANT

*BY SMART READS*

## Free Audiobook

As a thank you for being a Smart Reader you can choose 2 FREE audiobooks from audible.com. Simply sign up for free by visiting www.audibletrial.com/Travis to get your books.


## Visit:

www.smartreads.co/freebooks

to receive Smart Reads books for FREE


## Check us out on Instagram:

www.instagram.com/smart_readers

@smart_readers

# ABOUT SMARTREADS

Choose Smart Reads and get smart every time. Smart Reads sorts through all the best content and condenses the most helpful information into easily digestible chunks.

We design our books to be short, easy to read and highly informative. Leaving you with maximum understanding in the least amount of time.

Smart Reads aims to accelerate the spread of quality information so we've taken the copyright off everything we publish and donate our material directly to the public domain. You can read our uncopyright below.

We believe in paying it forward and donate 5% of our net sales to Pencils of Promise to build schools, train teachers and support child education.

To limit our footprint and restore forests around the globe we are planting a tree for every 10 hardcover books we sell.

Thanks for choosing Smart Reads and helping us help the planet.

Sincerely,

Travis & the Smart Reads Team

# TABLE OF CONTENTS

# INTRODUCTION

Cannabis is a controversial substance for many people. For some, cannabis brings on thoughts of good times and possibly getting "high." For others, especially today, it can bring hope of a medical cure or at the least, relief from a health condition they've been grappling with.

Whatever your thoughts are on the subject of cannabis, one thing is for sure: the cannabis plant is one of the most versatile and useful things in nature. It can be grown pretty much anywhere in any climate, either indoors or outside.

More and more, research and clinical trials are being conducted to find out information about cannabis and the wide array of health conditions it can potentially assist with.

Despite being illegal in many places for most of the last century, it is now being re-introduced into the mainstream society whereby not only medical cannabis has been made legal but recreational marijuana has been decriminalized in some countries and even in several states within the U.S.

This book is intended as a general guide to give you information about the history, the use and the medical potential of cannabis. It is our hope that this book helps you uncover some of the mysteries of cannabis and marijuana so please read on and enjoy.

# CHAPTER 1: WHAT IS CANNABIS?

Cannabis, also termed as marijuana, is a plant that's part of the Cannabaceae genus. There are three main species that are recognized but there are people who believe many more exist. The cannabis plant is grown around the world today, but is native to parts of central Asia including India. It is believed to have come from the mountainous Himalayas.

When it flowers annually, one major leaflet is the first to appear. Over time, this multiplies and each plant leaf can have a maximum of thirteen leaflets. However, the average number ranges from seven to nine pieces only. Cannabis plant flowers can be categorized as "female" or "male," with some plant capable of both.

One of the main reasons people grow cannabis is that they produce cannabinoids. This chemical group creates both physical as well as mental effects when it is ingested. The dried flower or bud form is then called resin or marijuana. In other countries, it's called hashish. However, during the start of last century, growing or even possessing cannabis became illegal in various portions of the world.

For a long time, cannabis has been used to make hemp fiber that can be used to make textiles. It can make hemp oil, which has potential medical use, and it can be used as what is termed a recreational drug. In recent years about 60,000 kilograms of cannabis were legally produced. In 2014, the estimated number of cannabis users was 182.5 million.

Cannabis is a popular recreational drug worldwide, coming only after alcohol, tobacco and caffeine. Different forms of the cannabis drug exist. These include extracts like hash oil and hashish. Many millions have used it. It is estimated that in the U.S. alone, more than 100 million Americans have tried cannabis. According to Delphic analysis done by British researchers in 2007, cannabis' risk factor for dependency is lower than alcohol and nicotine. Daily cannabis use, however, can sometimes cause psychological withdrawal symptoms like insomnia and irritability. Any withdrawal symptoms from cannabis use are often mild and not life threatening.

Marijuana can be consumed in many different ways. It can be rolled and made into a joint with rolling paper. Tobacco can be added into the mixture in order to provide extra flavor. This will also make the joints burn slower and is called a "spliff." Marijuana can also be smoked in cigar shells, which are referred to as "blunts."

Another way of smoking marijuana is by using a pipe. A bong is a type of pipe whereby smoke passes through water. This is regarded by some as a more effective way of reducing exposure to the carcinogens in cigarette smoke. Using it in a vaporizer is another way to use cannabis. A vaporizer will heat the cannabis and the active ingredients will be vaporized without burning the cannabis. This helps to eliminate some of the harmful effects of smoking, however, some studies have concluded it is just as bad.

Cannabis can also be eaten. It can also be steeped in tea, used in tinctures, and made into balms for hands and lips.

# CHAPTER 2: A BRIEF HISTORY OF CANNABIS

Cannabis cultivation can be traced back to around 12,000 years. This places the cannabis plant among the oldest cultivated crops in human history.

In many tropical or humid areas around the world, cannabis Sativa grows naturally. It was used as a mind-altering drug for many centuries, archaeologists finding evidence of this in Euro-Asian and African prehistoric societies. It has also been used for medicinal purposes for many centuries. There's evidence showing ancient Chinese cultures weaving hemp, wearing hemp clothing, and producing hemp pottery.

The use of cannabis in Egypt can be recorded as far back as 2,000 B.C. The information was found on scrolls that depicted medicinal plants. It was used to treat a range of physical ailments as well as sorrow and bad humor, in other words to help lift the mood and emotions of people. Cannabis pollen was found in the tomb of one of Egypt's most famous pharaohs, Rameses II and research has linked cannabis pollen to every royal mummy.

With regards to cannabis being mentioned in writing, some of the oldest records are from the Greek historian named Herodotus. He mentions cannabis being used in steam baths in central Eurasia by the Scythians, who are now modern day Iranians. In 440 BC, Herodotus wrote, "The Scythians, as I said, take some of this hemp-seed [presumably, flowers] and, creeping under the felt coverings, throw it upon the red-hot stones; immediately it smokes, and gives out such a vapor as no Grecian vapor-bath can exceed; the Scythes, delighted, shout for joy."

The ancient Greeks used cannabis for the treatment of nosebleeds, and also to expel tapeworms from the body. Not only did they use it on themselves but they also used cannabis on their animals, in particular their horses. They would immerse the seeds and the leaves in warm water then drink the juice. Cannabis sap was taken from immature plants and used for treating occlusion and easing blood circulation as well as ear infections. There is also evidence to suggest cannabis was used to treat gonorrhea. Cannabis seeds were also thrown into bonfires and the fumes were inhaled.

During their time in the Middle East, the ancient Greeks and the Romans used cannabis. Cannabis usage later spread throughout the Islamic Empire and into North Africa. It later reached the western hemisphere around 1545 and the Spaniards brought it to South

America (Chile) to use its fiber. It was later used in clothing, paper, and rope in North America.

There is also recorded history of cannabis use in China. The Emperor Shen Neng used it as medicine and at a later period hemp paper was made. In the Xinjiang Uyghur region of China a 2,700-year-old grave was discovered. It is the resting place of a shaman thought to be from the Jushi culture. At his head and by his feet were leather baskets within which were wooden bowls filled with cannabis. They were perfectly preserved. The archaeological team believes that the cannabis would have been used as a psychoactive agent, medicinally, or perhaps to aid divination.

Cannabis has had a rich and varied history in India, where it is called bhang. It is veiled in both legend and religion. It is mentioned as "sacred grass" in various religious texts. One of the earliest mentions of cannabis is found in the Hindu sacred texts referred to as The Vedas. It is believed this writing was compiled around 2,000 to 14,000 B.C. Cannabis is one of five sacred plants mentioned and according to the texts, an angel lives in the cannabis leaves.

The Vedas refers to cannabis as a joy-giver, a liberator, and a source of happiness. It was given to people in the pursuit of delight and happiness and to help them eliminate fear. One of the more famous Hindu gods, Shiva, is often associated with cannabis. In the Middle Ages, Indian soldiers would take a drink of bhang before battle; the same way westerners would often take a swig of whiskey.

Iran also has a history with cannabis and even today many people there use cannabis in the traditional manner. In the Zend Avesta, an ancient Persian religious text compiled around 559and 379 BCE, there is mention of "bhanga" or cannabis, as the "good narcotic." It is mentioned in the text several times as a means of achieving spiritual enlightenment. The famous Sufi mystic in Islam is also known to have used cannabis as a sacrament.

Another religious text that some believe mentions cannabis is the Talmud. It refers to the euphoriant properties of the cannabis plant in some sections and it is believed that hemp clothing and other accessories were made during that time in the region.
During Napoleon's travels through Egypt, he discovered that the lower classes there were habitually using hashish. When his soldiers returned to France, they brought this tradition back with them but when Napoleon found out he declared a prohibition.

Fast forward, many centuries where in 1800, marijuana plantations were flourishing in states like Georgia, South Carolina, Mississippi, California, and even up to New York. Smoking hashish became popular more so in France but caught on to a lesser extent in the U.S.

In 1890, marijuana and other cannabis products were made illegal and its importation banned into many countries. However, Queen Victoria's physician, Sir J.R. Reynolds prescribed her medicinal marijuana. He was influenced by the Irish doctor, William Brooke O'Shaughnessy, who invented the modern cholera treatment and pioneered the modern use of medical cannabis. O'Shaughnessy conducted clinical marijuana trials for illnesses such as hydrophobia, tetanus, convulsions, and rheumatism.

Queen Victoria's physician, Dr. Reynolds, prescribed cannabis to relieve menstrual cramping experienced by the monarch. He wrote, "When pure and administered carefully, [cannabis] is one of the most valuable medicines we possess." Only a few years after this, syringe usage became more widespread and due to its effectiveness of dissolving into patients' bloodstreams quickly, medical marijuana lost its popularity in Europe.

In 1928 in Geneva, the international drugs conference was held where cannabis was deemed to be as dangerous as opium and subsequently banned in the United Kingdom. In the U.S., cannabis was prohibited from 1915 onwards starting with the state of California, then Texas in 1919, Louisiana in 1924, and then New York in 1927.

In Asia, cannabis was still being grown and sold legally, however. In 1930's Chinese Turkestan, exports of 91,000 kilograms of hashish were sent to the northwestern frontiers of India. Legal and taxed hashish imports continue from Central Asia into India.

**An American History of Cannabis**

Cannabis has not always been illegal in the United States. The Puritans actually brought hemp with them to New England in 1645. Europeans were growing it even earlier in some South American nations. George Washington had hemp planted (among other things) on his estate on Mount Vernon. Thomas Jefferson would farm hemp and even brought seeds from China into the U.S. at risk of imprisonment.

Cannabis extract became a popular medicinal drug in the Americas during the 1800's. However, by the 1900's, its popularity began to turn. Mexican

immigrants then got associated with the smoked
version of marijuana by the 1920s. This eventually
fuelled the anti-immigrant feeling felt throughout the
U.S. and the move for prohibition began.

This went on until the 1930's and eventually cannabis
got banned in 24 states. Soon, the Federal Bureau of
Narcotics started a campaign against the drug. Media
sources sensationalized its effects, even aggravating
the situation. In 1937, the Marihuana Tax Act was
approved by the United States Congress. This banned
marijuana entirely save for just a few medicinal uses.
When the Second World War came, the U.S.
government promoted hemp and over a million acres
of land was used for planting because of the program.

In the 1950's, penalties were stiffened for marijuana
possession through the Narcotics Control Act and
Boggs Act. The penalty for first-time offenses was a
prison sentence between two to ten years as well as a
minimum fine of $20,000. In the 1970's the penalties
were relaxed a little but then in the 80's when Ronald
Reagan became president, penalties for marijuana
possession were once again raised. The Controlled
Substances Act was then regulated as a Schedule 1
drug, which meant that the U.S. government
considered it to have a high potential for abuse. It also

considered it to have no legitimate therapeutic or medicinal purposes.

Fast forward a few decades and cannabis is making a comeback. In the USA, the use of cannabis for medical purposes is now legal in 28 states. It is also legal in Guam and Puerto Rico. It all started in 1973 when Oregon liberalized cannabis laws through decriminalization. California was the first U.S. state to legalize medical cannabis and in 2012, Washington and Colorado legalized cannabis for recreational usage.

# CHAPTER 3: RECREATIONAL USE

Cannabis has been a popular recreational drug worldwide for some time now. Marijuana is the slang term for parts of the cannabis plant and it is what is mostly used as the recreational drug. Marijuana is also called weed, pot, ganja, mary Jane, and many other nicknames.

As already mentioned, it comes second only to alcohol, caffeine, and tobacco, which are also considered as having recreational usage. The most common forms of cannabis for recreational use are marijuana and hashish, which are either smoked or eaten.

Recreational drugs are used for their psychoactive effects to alter the mental state of the user. It modifies people's perceptions, emotions, and feelings.  When a recreational drug enters the body it will create an intoxicating effect, which is often called a "high." This is what many people who use these drugs are looking for.

Cannabis has psychoactive effects that are biphasic, meaning it has two different phases. The primary psychoactive effects generally include relaxation and in some cases euphoria, although this occurs to a much lesser extent. The secondary psychoactive effects include introspection and the facility to think philosophically. It also has a metacognition effect that is an awareness and understanding of one's thought processes. Other effects of cannabis can be hunger and an increased heart rate.

Regular cognition returns about three hours after taking cannabis in larger doses via bong smoking or vaporizing. If it is taken orally and in large amounts, the effects of the cannabis will last a lot longer, even up to a few days. This will also depend on one's tolerance to cannabis and the frequency of use.

It has been found that marijuana, as well as the illegal cocaine and ecstasy, have noticeable effects on sleep. Smoking marijuana or taking it orally reduces the REM sleep. Acute cannabis administration seems to facilitate falling asleep and increases Stage 4 sleep.

Cannabis in pretty much any form was illegal in the U.S. for decades. However, 26 states now have laws that legalize marijuana in some forms. More states will be joining these after they have passed measures allowing medical marijuana use. Seven District of Columbia states have more expansive laws that legalize recreational marijuana use.

Marijuana has been the most commonly used illicit drug in the U.S. and its use is widespread amongst younger people. Yearly surveys of middle and high school students have shown that marijuana usage has steadied in recent years after many years of increase. Adult recreational usage, as mentioned, has been legalized in some states. According to the 2012 National Survey on Drug Use and Health, 7.3% of Americans aged 12 years or older, had used marijuana within the previous 30 days. The average age of users when they first used it was 19 years old.

Usually people will hand roll cigarettes or use marijuana in water pipes, or bongs. More people are choosing to use vaporizers that pull the active ingredients, including THC, the main mind altering ingredient found in the cannabis plant. Sometimes, people like to mix marijuana in certain foods. They might add it to brownies, other cookies, or in tea.

Marijuana has both short and long term effects. Because it over-activates certain parts of the brain that have a higher numbers of receptors, it can cause the "high" that many people feel. Other effects are: altered senses such as seeing brighter colors, an altered sense of time, impaired body movements, mood changes, impaired memory, and difficulty thinking or problem solving.

Marijuana can also affect brain development in people who might have been using it as teenagers, for example. They may experience reduced memory and learning functions and it could affect the way the brain builds connections between areas that are necessary for learning and memory. People who started using marijuana as adults did not show any noticeable decline in these areas.

Most people who end up using cannabis want to experience relaxation and a mild sense of euphoria - the high. Cannabis will change the user's mood as well as affect how they perceive and think about their environment. When people are on recreational marijuana, everyday activities like listening to music or watching television can become altered, including becoming more intense.

The effects of cannabis can start within only a few minutes after inhaling and they can last for a few hours for cannabis plants that contain high levels of THC, the compound that gets people "high." If it is taken in food or liquid, the effects will be felt longer.

As mentioned, cannabis has both short-term and long-term effects. The short-term effects can include:
• Feelings of well-being

- Drowsiness
- Talkativeness
- Loss of inhibitions
- Increased appetite
- Decreased nausea
- Loss of coordination
- Bloodshot eyes
- Paranoia
- Dry eyes, mouth and throat

There can also be some side effects such as short-term memory lapses, impaired motor skills, red eyes, or feeling anxious or paranoid. It has also been found that children whose mothers used cannabis during pregnancy may have behavioral problems. This might also be the case for people who started smoking marijuana at a younger age i.e. in their teens.

The long-term effects can include:
- Decreased memory and learning abilities
- Decreased motivation
- An increased risk of respiratory illnesses associated with smoking.

The leaves, flower buds, and stem extracts from the marijuana plant can be vaporized, brewed in tea or put into tinctures. They can also be placed in food and eaten. There are literally hundreds of compounds found in marijuana but the one responsible for the drug's psychoactive effects is tetrahydrocannbinol, or THC as already mentioned.

It is THC that binds to cannabinoid receptors throughout the human body. The "high" from marijuana comes from the THC binding to certain brain regions that are responsible for pleasure, pain, and perception. This information is taken from the National Institute on Drug Abuse (NDA).

Going by the United States Department of Health, there are around 400,000 emergency room visits associated with cannabis use. This, however, is a little misleading due to the fact that the statistics include visits whereby patients were treated for conditions where cannabis was implicated but was not necessarily the direct cause of the emergency room visit. Most illicit drug hospital visits actually involve multiple drugs. It is also important to note that marijuana bought on the streets has often been tampered with, meaning other chemicals including hair spray and/or glass powder have been added in order to make it seem like the buds are densely covered and to make the marijuana heavier so the dealers can charge more per gram.

Purchasing cannabis illegally means people run the risk of getting untested cannabis which has been contaminated, not only with the elements mentioned in the above paragraph but also with PCP, also known as angel dust. This is a dissociative drug and can bring on hallucinations and/or violent episodes. It is clear then, that illegally bought cannabis can be very dangerous and is definitely not recommended. The manner in which the illegally bought cannabis strains have been added to has nothing to do with the actual plant itself.

# CHAPTER 4: INDUSTRIAL HEMP

Hemp is the common name for plants of the entire genus Cannabis. Hemp is generally the term used only in reference to cannabis strains, which are cultivated for industrial usages and non-recreational use.

Cannabis is a hearty type of plant that can grow up to 18 feet tall in a short amount of time. It can pop up along the side of the road or driveways from stray seeds. Cannabis, which is grown for industry, is called industrial hemp and sometimes-industrial marijuana.

Industrial hemp is used for many things such as paper, biodegradable plastics, textiles, rope, health food, fuel, and some construction products. It can also be crushed and used for food and even beauty products. It is one of the earliest domesticated plants and a fast growing biomass, an organic matter used as fuel, especially in power stations. It is also one of the Green Future objectives, which are now growing in popularity as more and more people become aware of renewable power and biodegradable products. The hemp plant does not require pesticides and does not cause topsoil erosion. It also produces oxygen.

In addition, hemp can be used as a replacement for many harmful products like tree paper, which uses a process of chlorine bleach resulting in toxic waste products that are carcinogenic, not to mention the deforestation that occurs. Hemp also produces four times more raw materials than trees for paper making and can be planted not only once, but up to three times in one season. This depends on the location of course. It can also be recycled around ten times. Wood pulp paper can only be recycled around three times.

It is estimated that each day around 48-56 thousand square miles of rainforest is lost. This works out to around one acre every few seconds. This is something very difficult to fathom. Many species will also be lost. It is not difficult to see how cannabis hemp would be of benefit to the earth.

Hemp can also be a replacement for some cosmetics and plastics that are mostly petroleum based and therefore do not decompose easily. With hemp, the strongest chemical necessary for whitening hemp paper is hydrogen peroxide, and this is not toxic. Just from these few examples it is easy to see that cannabis has many positives.

Many countries worldwide produce industrial hemp. Some of the biggest producers are Canada, China, and France. Hemp is exported from other nations into the U.S. in larger amounts than any other nation, as current U.S. law prohibits hemp farming with only a few exceptions.

Hemp can be organically grown on most farmlands around the world. Many varieties exist and they can be chosen for their various characteristics. For example, some may be chosen for their high oil content, others for the length of their fibers. Seed banks hold more than one hundred industrial hemp stains.

The hemp plant itself grows rapidly, maturing in 8 to 12 weeks' time after planting. It has a strong resistance to most plant pests, and will choke out weeds around it. The hemp plant also has long roots that are able to reach water deep into the earth. They bind and aerate the soil in places where other plants cannot, and hemp crops can be used for reclaiming land in certain areas such as those prone to drought or flooding.

When the hemp plant is ready for harvesting it will provide a high cellulose yield, oils, edible proteins, and fibers that can be used for literally thousands of product applications across many different industries. Due to hemp's versatility, a famine-stricken village would be able to house, feed, and clothe itself just from one hemp field. Hemp therefore, represents a real lifeline crop.

Before the 1880's, around 90% of the world's paper was actually made from cannabis hemp. Some important historical documents were written on hemp paper. These include two drafts of the U.S. Declaration of Independence, and the Gutenberg Bible.

**More Interesting Information about Hemp**

• Fabrics made from at least 50% hemp will block out the sun's harmful UV rays more effectively than other fabrics.

• School textbooks were crafted from flax paper and hemp up until the 1880s rolled in.

• In America, it was legal for people to pay taxes using hemp. This was the case from around 1631 until the early 1800's.

• President Washington grew hemp.

• Americans were legally bound to grow hemp during the Colonial Era and the Early Republic.

• Henry Ford's first Model T could run on hemp as well as gasoline.

# CHAPTER 5: CANNABIS AROUND THE WORLD

Every country has its own laws and regulations regarding cannabis, both the recreational kind and the medicinal kind. For travelers, making themselves aware of the laws of the land is a must. Cannabis possession, use and dealing are criminalized in most countries. However, in many countries where it's legal, there are certain conditions placed including how much an individual should have at any given time.

Cannabis is completely legal in only a couple of nations without any restrictions.
For example, people mistakenly believe marijuana is legal in the Netherlands. This is, in fact, not correct. Indeed, Holland is famous for having a tolerant drug policy and a lot of people don't realize that drugs are illegal there. Understanding the Dutch drug policy can spare travelers a lot of trouble.

It is illegal to produce, sell, possess, import or export drugs in Holland. The government, however, has created a drug policy that tolerates cannabis smoking under strict conditions and terms. Coffee shops, for example, can sell soft drugs to customers but no more than five grams of cannabis per person per day. All coffee shops must adhere to strict laws and adhere to the legal amount of soft drugs and the conditions in which they are sold and used. They cannot advertise drugs or sell them to under 18's.

For some people, the laws and the reality of drug use in Holland might seem contradictory. The Dutch government recognizes it is impossible to prevent people from using drugs. Therefore, coffee shops can legally sell only small amounts and only soft drugs. This is seen as a more pragmatic approach and means the Dutch authorities can focus on catching bigger criminals who make large profits from drugs or those who push hard drugs.

In Portugal, there were changes to the law, which meant consumption, or possession of all illegal drugs in small quantities was decriminalized. This means possession of personal quantities of drugs, including cannabis, is not considered a crime. It might surprise some to find that since this law was passed, Portugal has experienced enormous benefits including a significant drop in the use of hard drugs. It is, however, illegal to cultivate cannabis, even in smaller amounts even if it could be considered for personal use.

In Australia, cannabis is the most widely used illicit drug with around 33% of Australians aged 22 or older having tried it. Medical cannabis is now being produced with some states making it legal to use and other states and territories considering changing legislation. However, each state has strict regulations, including what illnesses medical cannabis can be used for. In the state of Victoria, for example, cannabis can be used by children with severe epilepsy but not for other conditions. This is correct at the time of writing this book.

Changes, which took place in November 2016, came through the Therapeutic Goods Administration. This means that medical cannabis will not fall under Australia's stringent schedules, which are reserved for the most dangerous drugs. There are provisions being put into place so it can be used for medical purposes. It is still illegal, however, to grow marijuana or use it for recreational purposes in Australia.

Meanwhile, it is completely legal in Uruguay so long as you are 18 years of age or over. In Argentina, it is legal to smoke cannabis in your own home but it is illegal to cultivate it or sell it.

In Iran, they have some seemingly contradictory cannabis laws. Both use and possession are almost entirely decriminalized, however, trafficking and dealing is harshly punished. In some cases, possession of flowering tops might be punishable and people could get a fine, but it must first be proven there was an intent to produce narcotic drugs in such cases. Iran has a big problem with drugs but drug addicts found possessing less than a gram of cannabis are exempt from any punishment. Growing cannabis, as long as it is not for producing narcotics, is not always penalized.

For anyone trafficking or dealing cannabis in any amount higher than 5 kilograms, the death penalty applies in Iran. For dealing or trafficking fifty grams or even less, fifty lashes is the punishment. The Iranian government is severely clamping down on drug trafficking due to the increase in stronger drugs such as opium and heroin being brought into and through the country in recent years.

In some countries in South East Asia, cannabis laws are quite relaxed. Cambodia has the most lenient laws regarding cannabis. The laws regarding marijuana are mostly in a grey area and cannabis violations are not a priority for the government.

Technically, Myanmar is not a marijuana friendly country and violations can get people a five to ten year sentence for possession. It is rare, however, that arrests are made for breaking marijuana laws. Myanmar has a big problem with opiates and the government focuses more on those.

Sometimes, the laws can be a little confusing and it is always recommended that if you are travelling overseas, you never just take a guess at what the laws may be in another country. Always check your information carefully. Use government websites and do your research well.

As most people already know, in some countries even a small amount of cannabis can get you arrested. In other nations the death penalty applies for certain drugs. This is why it's important to always research and know the laws whenever you are travelling.

# CHAPTER 6: THE MAIN DIFFERENCE BETWEEN HEMP AND MARIJUANA

Both hemp and marijuana are two popular names for the cannabis plant. Often, cannabis is associated with the marijuana drug and getting high as well as durable paper, military grade fabric, and plant-based plastics. In reality, hemp and marijuana have their differences. So how are they different? There are five main aspects of the plants that make them differ:

1. **Genetics** – As mentioned in a previous chapter, cannabis is thought to be one of the oldest domesticated crops grown by humans. Throughout history, people have used different types of cannabis for both medicinal and industrial uses.

Early civilizations grew the tall, sturdy type of plants to make oils, foods, and textiles such as fabric and rope. The plants they grew were bred with other plants, which had the same type of characteristics, and this led to the cannabis type known as hemp.

Other cannabis plants were known for their psychoactive properties and were selectively bred for medical purposes. They were also used for certain religious purposes. This led to the variety of cannabis plant now known as marijuana.

The main agricultural differences between cannabis and hemp are mostly in their genetic parentage and the cultivation environment. Scientists believe the earlier separation of the cannabis plant genes led to two very distinct cannabis plants. These species are identified as Cannabis Indica and Cannabis Sativa.

2. **Cultivation** – Both marijuana and hemp are farmed for different reasons. Due to this fact, they need different types of growing conditions.

Medicinal cannabis has been bred selectively over time and the characteristics it contains are optimized through its specific cultivation environment. This will produce female flowering plants that will produce budding flowers at the flowering stage of their life cycle.

On the other hand, hemp plants are mostly male and don't have flowering buds during their life cycle. Over many centuries of selective breeding, low THC content and fast growing cannabis plants have been cultivated.

For those who want to grow marijuana with high THC levels it can be a little tricky because it needs close attention and specific room conditions. It will need stable temperatures, stable lighting and the right amount of humidity and oxygen levels. Hemp on the other hand, can easily be grown outdoors and usually is, which maximizes the yield and the size. It does not require so much attention either.

3. **The Legality** - Despite certain types of cannabis being illegal in many countries there are around thirty others where hemp is grown. Some of the top hemp producing nations in the world is China, the European Union and now Canada. Around $500 million worth of hemp products are imported into the United States yearly.

Marijuana is still illegal throughout most of the world with the exception of some legislation as mentioned in previous chapters. It is still considered a narcotic and so legal marijuana production is subject to strict rules, more so than hemp. However, medical marijuana is being researched in more and more countries and, under strict rules, it is also being used on patients.

4. **Composition** – All cannabis plants contain certain unique compounds that are called cannabinoids. Through recent research it has been found that over 60 different cannabinoids exist that are known so far. THC is probably the one that is most well known, probably because it's the one that creates the "high."

In contrast, hemp plants contain little THC. This is what most people rely on to help them distinguish between marijuana and hemp. The Canadian government, for example, has a maximum THC level in a cannabis plant at 0.3% and anything higher than that is considered to be marijuana.

Now, medical marijuana, on the other hand, can produce THC levels between 5 to 20% as an average. Some medical marijuana plants can even have 25 to 30% THC. Both hemp and marijuana contain the important CBD compound. Hemp plants have more CBD than they do THC and marijuana obviously, has more THC than it does CBD. It is also known that the CBD compound reduces the psychoactive effects of the THC compound, another difference between the plants.

5. **Research** – Both marijuana and hemp cannabis are subject to strict laws and this can, and often does, make research somewhat difficult. Within the United States and Canada alone, there are thousands of organizations, both academic and research types, that are equipped enough to perform either medical or agricultural research in cannabis, but only about forty of them have the right type of research license to be able to study cannabis, even in a limited capacity. Even though these barriers exist, researchers are still

making quite a bit of progress and are better understanding the way that medical marijuana can work to help manage different illnesses or disorders.

Research is also providing us with more information about how the hemp plant can contribute to society and the future in positive ways, not just medicinally but also environmentally. For example, the University of Alberta researchers recently developed a supercapacitor using raw hemp. This has made the possibility of manufacturing fast-charging, cheap batteries real. Hemp fiber has also been used to make new types of plastic and because of this it is becoming a commonly used material in car production.

As the legalization of cannabis begins to spread around the world, newer opportunities will become available to explore cannabis' potential for both hemp and marijuana.

# CHAPTER 7: MEDICAL CANNABIS

Cannabis and medical marijuana contain many medical benefits as has been discovered recently. Cannabis' reputation has been rising with increasing positive results taken from researchers about the cannabinoids.

CBD is short for cannabidiol, a compound found in the well-known and once illicit cannabis as well as the legal industrial component of cannabis, which is called hemp. The CBD compound has significant medical benefits without getting the "high" part of it. It is only in recent years that cannabis, CBD and THC have seen some positive media attention, and this attention has removed the stigma of it being an illegal Schedule I drug.

Marijuana legalization has become a hot topic in the last few years, especially as many states in the U.S. approved the use of medical marijuana. In some states, recreational marijuana usage has also been approved. Medical cannabis is also legal in many other countries worldwide and is becoming more and more accepted for its medicinal properties.

**Facts About CBD**

In cannabis, CBD is considered the major ingredient. Cannabis contains a huge number of compounds, often belonging to the cannabinoid group of molecules. Both THC and CBD are usually found in higher concentrations compared to the others, hence, the focus of most studies is on these two.

Different cannabis plants will have differing levels of CBD and THC. For example, marijuana specifically grown for recreational purposes will contain more THC than it does CBD. By using certain breeding techniques, however, cannabis breeders have now created cannabis varieties with higher levels of CBD and close to zero levels of THC. These have become a lot more popular recently.

As for CBD, this has been shown to have no psychoactive assets. It doesn't have the capacity to get people high and is therefore studied for its possible advantage as medication. This also makes it a poor choice for recreational marijuana users.

A study conducted and published on the 2011 Current Drug Safety, stated that CBD doesn't have any bearing on psychomotor and psychological functions when ingested.  They also deemed that CBD is "well

tolerated and safe" even when used in higher doses
during treatment.

A review done in 2013 and was subsequently
published on the British Journal of Clinical
Pharmacology stated that CBD has many medicinal
benefits. This included:

- Anti-depressant
- Antipsychotic properties
- Anti-inflammatory
- Anticonvulsant
- Anti-tumoral and anti-cancer
- Antioxidant
- Antiemetic (prevents nausea and vomiting)

The information for the research was taken from
studies done on animals but more clinical tests today
are being done on humans. A leading UK company has
even announced that they're studying the effects of
CBD as a possible treatment for forms of
schizophrenia and epilepsy. While another medical
center in California is looking at CBD to help treat
breast cancer.

What's more, it's been shown that CBD helps minimize
the effects of THC. At this point, it seems to have

resistant properties to THC, acting as a natural barrier to the "high" that THC produces. Although both THC and CBD do not produce a lethal threat when taken in high doses, the side effects can be prevented when taking cannabis with only high CBD levels.

# CHAPTER 8: CANNABIS AND GROWING ENVIRONMENTS

**Growing Cannabis Indoors**

Since marijuana is becoming legal or being decriminalized in many countries including a number of U.S. states, growing cannabis is becoming more popular. Indoor hydroponic systems are now easier to work with and they can produce good yields.

Ventilation is also important when growing cannabis indoors. The right type of ventilation cannot is crucial in grow rooms because cannabis plants constantly need carbon dioxide. The air must be circulated and supplied consistently then removed when it becomes stale. Appropriate ventilation can help minimize any bad odors.

Sometimes, plant odors can be strong in grow rooms and air fresheners will not be appropriate to get rid of them. In such cases, ozone generators can be utilized and they will curb the plant odors drastically. Ozone generators work but they can get expensive and need further construction. Meanwhile, carbon filters hooked up to the exhaust fans can also stop plant odors. The way they work is, they sift odors through the charcoal in the filters and expel the stale, odorous air. Carbon filters are faster to install and also easier to use compared to ozone generators.

Fans are also used to replace wind. The wind is necessary because it stirs the stalks and leaves which ensures they grow stronger. It also helps to ward of bug pests and dust. Fans are necessary, however, they are not useful in curbing plant odors.

The temperature in grow rooms must be maintained at certain levels. The ideal level for grow rooms is between 70 to 85 degrees Fahrenheit, or between 20 to 30 degrees Celsius. Lighting will produce heat and the vents and fans also affect the room temperature. The season outside will also have an effect on whether the room temperature will rise or drop. Of course, summer is always the hottest.

Diseases and pests are another consideration. Poor ventilation and temperatures as well as humidity will make for the growth of spider mites. Fans that oscillate and a temperature of 75 degrees will help to ward off many insect pests.

Considering all these things, it is easy to see that growing cannabis indoors can be quite complex and many considerations need to be applied. However, grow rooms also have advantages including security.

**Growing Cannabis Outdoors**

For those who prefer to grow cannabis outdoors as it has originally been for thousands of years, the information below can help to give an idea of how it can be done. It must be stressed, however, that you must be sure it is legal in the area in which you live.

Some of you might think that, in order to grow your own cannabis outdoors, it is necessary to be in a hot or sub-tropical climate. This is not the case. Cannabis can be grown in hot climates as well as the type of climate found in the far north of America and Europe, including Alaska and the Scandinavian nations. Nature has provided the cannabis plant with strength and a way of adapting so that it can grow in many different regions.

However, the right site for growing outdoors must be chosen carefully. To choose a potential growing site you must think about the most basic requirements that a marijuana plant needs as well as whether the site can be accessed easily. It's probably a good idea to ensure cannabis plants are also hidden from view for a range of different reasons.

Marijuana can still be a contentious issue for some people, perhaps some neighbors. It is also a good idea to be discrete in case of theft.

Cannabis grown in the woods is best keep far away from walking tracks or paths. Look out for hikers and dog walkers as well as signs of passing.

Something that must be carefully considered is if the area offers the plants all the natural requirements, the most important of course, being sunlight. The more sunlight the plants get, the more they will grow. The minimum amount of sunlight that cannabis plants need to grow is 6 hours per day.

It would be beneficial if the plants could get more than six hours. The plants are best grown in areas where they won't be shaded over by other plants. So, unrestricted sunlight for as much of the day as possible is a must. Internet maps and local knowledge can be used to find the best places to plant.

Cannabis requires large amounts of water to thrive. In areas where the climate naturally has high rainfall it will be better. In areas with little rainfall, the irrigation systems must be good. The proper amount of water is crucial to the cannabis plant.

Cannabis also needs good soil, the type that will compact when it's squeezed and not break apart. Clay or rocky soil will not do. It must also have a good pH levels, the ideal being around 5.5 to 6.5. The soil must be well drained in order to avoid patches of standing water.

# CHAPTER 9: CANNABIS OIL

Cannabis oil is its own entity when discussing the use of cannabis for recreational purposes, or cannabis extracts for use within the medical area. Oil that has been extracted from the cannabis plant is a concentrated mixture of the components within cannabis. It is already recognized as a treatment for conditions such as cancer, and other chronic illnesses.

Cannabis has been the subject of extensive medical research recently. There are many different types of cannabis strains and different elements in each that will react in different ways when placed in different conditions and/or environments. This is why it is highly recommended that those thinking about making their own cannabis oil take the time to research carefully before embarking on producing it.

The product made will only be as effective as the time and effort taken to choose the right production method. Another thing to remember if you decide to make your own cannabis oil is that every compound will only be effective in treating a select number of medical conditions. You must put in the time and effort to research which combinations are best for the condition you are looking to ease. If this is done, you should be able to produce effective remedies. It might be a good idea to use organic cannabis that has not been affected with insecticides, pesticides, or chemical fertilizers as this can affect an individual with a poor or already compromised immune function.

It is important to know certain terms such as THC and CBD. It will be necessary to know exactly what they stand for. These have been mentioned in earlier chapters. It is these compounds that have an effect on the brain and body. It is what gives people the "high" when it is smoked or taken orally (as in food).

On the other hand, CBD is short for cannabidiol. It is a compound also found in the legal industrial component of cannabis - hemp. It is this CBD compound which has quite a lot to offer. The CBD compound has significant medical benefits without getting the "high" part of it. It is only in recent years that cannabis, CBD and THC have seen positive media attention and this attention has removed the stigma of it being an illegal Schedule I drug.

Marijuana legalization has become a hot topic in the last few years, especially as twenty-nine states in the U.S. approved the use of medical marijuana. In eight different states, recreational marijuana usage has also been approved.

The combination of oils rich in CBD and THC are thought to assist with certain illnesses. They are, however, less effective than the combinations that contain high CBD and low THC. Chemical compounds that contain elements from other plants as well as cannabis also seem to be more effective than the compounds that only contain cannabis plant extracts. For anyone who is thinking about using cannabis oil for the treatment of any condition, it is advised that they seek the help of a health professional. This is very important and is not something to mess around with.

Diseases that are thought to benefit from cannabis oil include:

- Anorexia
- Obesity
- Glaucoma
- Cancer
- Chronic pain
- Epilepsy
- Heart disease
- Multiple Sclerosis
- Osteoporosis
- Schizophrenia
- Anxiety and Stress
- Metabolic syndrome-related disorders

As you can see, it is a versatile oil, however, it is also important to note that research and detailed information on cannabis and its potential health benefits is still in the infancy stage. It is also important to advise readers that others who are looking to make a quick buck have scammed some people. If you are thinking of purchasing cannabis for medicinal purposes, it is imperative that you buy from reputable companies and not some webpage you found on the Internet. It is also necessary to check with your doctor.

Hemp oil is obtained by pressing the benefit-rich hemp seeds and is a little different to cannabis oil, even though they both come from the same genus and also the same species that is cannabis sativa. Hemp is the term used for a cannabis sativa plant that only contains small amounts of THC.

Cannabis oil is a concentrated and distilled form of marijuana. All the plant material is stripped away using a solvent. It can be used with other oils and also used to make a variety of edible cannabis-infused foods.

**Cannabis Oil Extraction**
A cannabis concentrate, also called cannabis extract, is a lot more potent than the standard cannabis buds. It has been used as an effective medicine for different

ailments and conditions. Cannabis extracts will be similar to the particular strain they were extracted from including having a similar taste and smell.

Due to the fact that cannabis is hydroponic, it will dissolve in water. In order to extract the healing properties of cannabis, particular solvents and oils would need to be used to break it down. The most commonly used solvents are alcohol that is 99% isopropyl, ethanol, coconut and olive oils. The extract that comes from this process is called cannabis oil, weed oil, marijuana oil or hash oil.

Cannabis extraction is complex and can be potentially dangerous due to the highly volatile and flammable solvents that must be used. Trained professionals can go through the process and are well prepared to do so.

Cannabis extraction can be done using Co2, which is of course, carbon dioxide. It is used under high pressure but low temperatures in order to isolate and preserve the purity of the oil.

As mentioned above, ethanol can also be used. High grain alcohol will create high quality cannabis oil. The only thing with this method is that it will destroy the plant waxes that may contain certain health benefits. Some producers of cannabis oil favor these waxes.

Another ingredient that can be used is olive oil. It is best to use extra virgin olive oil but regular olive oil will do as well. This particular method is considered both inexpensive and safe, as there is little chance of olive oil blowing up. The only thing to watch out for with this method is that it is perishable and must be stored in a cool, dark place.

# CONCLUSION

It is clear going by the information provided in this book (and perhaps research you might decide to do on your own), that the cannabis plant is indeed a useful and versatile plant. It does deserve a lot more research in order to find out the full potential that it can provide to humans and the planet. Its uses are numerous and are not only confined to medicine as has been shown by the many uses hemp provides. The possibilities seem to be enormous and scientists and medical professionals are taking a closer look at the cannabis plant.

# THANKS FOR READING

We really hope you enjoyed this book. If you found this material helpful feel free to share it with friends. You can also help others find it by leaving a review where you purchased the book. Your feedback will help us continue to write books you love.

The Smart Reads library is growing by the day! Make sure and check out the other wonderful books in our catalog. We would love to hear which books are your favorite.

# SMART READS ORIGINS

Smart Reads was born out of the desire to find the best information fast without having to wade through the sheer volume of fluff available online. Smart Reads combs through massive amounts of knowledge compiles the best into quick to read books on a variety of subjects.

We consider ourselves Smart Readers, not dummies. We know reading is smart. We're self taught. We like to learn a TON about a WIDE variety of topics. We have developed a love for books and we find intelligence attractive.

We found that each new topic we tried to learn about started with the challenge of finding the pieces of the puzzle that mattered most. It becomes a treasure hunt rather than an education.

Smart Reads wants to find the best of the best information for you. To condense it into a package that you can consume in an hour or less.  So you can read more books about more topics in less time.

# OUR MISSION

Smart Reads aims to accelerate the availability of useful information and will publish a high quality book on every major topic on amazon.

Smart Reads hopes to remove barriers to sharing by taking the copyright off everything we publish and donating it to the public domain. We hope other publishers and authors will follow our example.

Our goal is to donate $1,000,000 or more by 2020 to build over 2,000 schools by giving 5% of our net profit to Pencils of Promise.

We want to restore forests around the globe by planting a tree for every 10 physical books we sell and hope to plant over 100,000 trees by 2020.

Doesn't it feel good knowing that by educating yourself you are helping the world be a better place? We think so too...

Thanks for helping us help the world. You Smart Reader you...

Travis and the Smart Reads Team

# WHY I STARTED SMART READS

Every time I wanted to learn about something new I'd have to buy 20 books on the topic and spend way too long sorting through them and reading them all until I arrived at the big picture. Until I had enough perspectives to know who was just guessing, who was uninformed and who had stumbled upon something remarkable.

I wished someone else could just go in and figure that out for me and tell me what matters. That's how smart reads was born. I want smart reads to be a company that does all that research up front. Sorts through all the content that is available on each topic and pulls out the most up to date complete understanding, then have people smarter than me package the best wisdom in an easy to understand way in the least amount of words possible.

For example, I got a new puppy so I wanted to learn about dog training. I bought 14 different books about dog training and by the time I got through the first 5 and finally started getting the big picture on the best way to train my puppy she had grown up into a dog.

Yeah she's well behaved. She doesn't poop in the house. I can get her to sit and come when I call. But what if someone else went in and read all those books for me, found the underlying themes and picked out the best information that would give me the big picture and get me right to the point. And I'd only have to read one book instead of 15.

That would be amazing. I would save time. And maybe
my dog would be rolling over, cleaning up after my
kids and doing the dishes by now. That my friend, is
the reason I started smart reads. Because I wanted a
company I can trust to deliver me the best information
in an easy to understand way that I can digest in under
an hour. Because dog training is one of many subjects I
want to master.

The quicker I can learn a wide variety of topics the
sooner that information can begin playing a role in
shaping my future. And none of us knows how long
that future will be. So why not do everything we can to
make the best of it and consume a ton of knowledge.
And I figured all the better if I can also make a positive
difference in the world.

That's why we're also building schools, planting trees
and challenging ideas about copyright's place in
today's world.  Because as a company we have to be
doing everything we can to support the ecosystem
that gives us all these beautiful places to read our
books. Thanks for reading.

Travis

# Customers Who Bought This

# Customers Who Bought This Book Also Bought

The Cannabis Pharmacy: Grow Cannabis, Make Hemp Oil and Know the Difference Between THC, CBD and the Medical Benefits of Cannabinoids

The Powerful Benefits of Myrrh: Effective Myrrh Recipes For Healthy & Beauty, Oil Pulling Therapy, Creativity, Aromatherapy and Improving The Mind

Beginner Gardening: Growing Vegetables and Ornamentals

Mint As Medicine: Discover The Powerful Healing Properties of Herb in Treating Headaches, Allergies, Asthma, Clarity and Peace of Mind

Probiotic Dieting: The Miracle of Probiotics in Healing Your Gut, Trimming Belly Fat and Weight Loss

Growing Cannabis: How to Cultivate and Make Your Own Cannabis Garden

MDMA and Other Psychedelic Drugs: Learning the Therapeutic Effects of LSD, Psilocybin and Other Mind-Bending Drugs